contents

RAPID 800 dinner

RAPID

800

COOKBOOK

QUICK AND SIMPLE RAPID **800** COOKBOOK
Lose Weight Fast

ISBN 978-1-913005-48-1

DISCLAIMER

Quick and simple - *lose weight fast.*

Rapid 800 = Delicious Dieting

So you're interested in 'fasting' but you still want to eat tasty, low calorie, healthy meals that taste delicious .Then welcome to the **Quick and Simple Rapid 800 Cookbook**. Filling calorie counted breakfasts to kick-start your day, fuss-free fast day lunches and flavour filled dinners all under 300, 500 and 800 calories.

Each of our tasty recipes are delicious, healthy, simple to make, guilt free and perfect when following the Rapid 800 Diet.

Intermittent fasting is a great and flexible way to approach weight loss and less restrictive that many other diets. Choice and taste are paramount when eating low calorie dishes so we've put together a wonderful selection of meals that are tasty, nutritious and most can be prepared and cooked in less than 30 minutes.

Imagine a diet where you can eat whatever you want for 5 days a week and fast for 2. That's what the 5:2 Diet is, and it's revolutionised the way people think about dieting. By allowing you the freedom to eat normally for MOST of the week and fast by restricting your calorie intake for just TWO non-consecutive days a week (800 calories per day for men and women), you keep yourself motivated and remove that dreaded feeling of constantly denying yourself the food you really want to eat.

It still takes willpower, but it's nowhere near as much of a grind when you know that you have tomorrow to look forward to. It's all about freedom. The ability to be flexible with the days you choose to fast makes the likelihood of you sticking to the diet for a prolonged period, or even indefinitely as a lifestyle choice, much higher than a regime that requires calorie restriction every single day.

Popularised by Dr. Michael J. Mosley, the 5:2 diet plan has been adopted as a way of life, which could change your relationship with dieting and weight loss.

What's more, this way of eating is believed to have major health benefits, which could alter your health forever!

Initially, back in 2012 the 5:2 Diet was based on a 500 calorie limit on fast days. Since then further research and knowledge has grown into how fasting can help with weight loss and as such a newer approach of 800 calories on fast days is recommended – especially for those who have already tried the 5:2 Diet but may have struggled to stick to 500 calories on their fast days. This new calorie limit represents a more manageable approach to dieting while still seeing results. It may take a little longer to lose weight compared to the 500 calorie option but the positive aspect is that you are more likely to stick to the plan long term, as it is less restrictive.

It's important to remember what exactly a calorie is when controlling the number we consume.

- **A calorie is a unit of energy.**

Scientifically, 1 calorie is the amount of energy required to raise one gram of water by one degree Celsius. To you and me, a calorie (a unit of energy) is a vital component of our body and its health. We need energy to go about our every day tasks and for our body to function and repair itself as it should. So energy (calories) are a necessity and are present in everything we eat – carbohydrates, protein and fat. We know that excess calories are linked to weight gain and poor health so maintaining a healthy level of calories or reducing calories to accelerate weight loss should be managed carefully and safely.

Aside from the increased calories, the other difference between the original 500 calorie option and the new 800 rule is the period of actual fasting. On the 800 plan you should include a 14 hour fast period either directly after your fast day or directly before your fast day.

So for example if you choose Monday as a fast day you might have an evening meal on Sunday at 6pm then completely fast until breakfast on Monday morning at 8am.

Alternatively fast for 14 hours following your last meal on your fast day. e.g. dinner at 5pm with breakfast on Tuesday at 7am.

Flexibility is the great thing about the 5:2 Diet but remember your fast days should be on 2 non-consecutive days and you must fast for a 14 hour period either before or after.

On your non-fast days, you can eat 'normally' without counting calories but try to follow a healthy diet – a Mediterranean approach is recommended with plenty of fish, salad, grains and nuts. You should enjoy your non-fast days but don't binge! Avoid processed food, snacking between meals and the usual temptations like fizzy drinks, biscuits, crisps, chocolate and alcohol.

how it works

The concept of fasting is an ancient one and modern science is uncovering evidence that fasting can be an extremely healthy way to shed extra weight. Research has shown that it can reduce levels of IGF-1 (insulin-like growth factor 1, which leads to accelerated ageing), activate DNA repair genes, and reduce blood pressure, cholesterol and glucose levels as well as suggestions of a lower risk of heart disease and cancers.

Fasting works by restricting your body to fewer calories than it uses. Most importantly, it does this in a way which remains healthy and is balanced by eating normally for the other 5 days of the week.

This book has been developed specifically to help you prepare your fast day meals, however if you want to find out more about the specific details of the science behind the fasting we recommend studying Dr. Michael J. Mosley's work and, as with all diets, you should consider seeking advice from a health professional before starting.

If you are pregnant, breastfeeding, diabetic, suffer from any eating disorder or are under the age of 18 we do not recommend this diet for you. If you suffer from any health issues you should first seek the advice of a health professional before embarking on any form of diet.

what will this book do for me?

This book will give you a wide choice of delicious, low calorie, easy to prepare meals that will not only form the basis of your 800 calorie fast plan but will also open your eyes to a new lifestyle choice which will help you lose weight and improve your overall health and immune system.

This book has been designed to provide a wide selection of easy to prepare recipes to keep you motivated and your engine stoked during your fasting day and, because you can eat normally for the 5 days a week, you'll be much more likely to stick with it over time and enjoy the long term health and weight benefits.

when can i expect to see results?

By the end of your first week in most cases! Obviously everybody is different, but where someone is carrying extra weight they will normally see a reduction in the first week of embarking on fasting. Typically many will see a greater weight loss at the beginning, followed by a slowing down then eventually settling around a stable healthy weight.

taking it week by week

The Rapid 800 can work for you whatever your lifestyle. Each week you should think carefully about which days are likely to be best suited to your fasting days and then stick with it (remembering to factor in your 14 hour fast period).

You can change your fast days each week or keep in a regular routine, whichever suits you best. Ideally your fasting days should be non-consecutive. This gives you the opportunity to stay motivated by eating normally the following day, although it can be acceptable to fast for 2 days consecutively if you are feeling particularly inspired.

Of course, reducing your calorie intake for two days will take some getting used to and inevitably there will be hunger pangs to start with, but you'll be amazed at how quickly your body adapts to your new style of eating.

how will i manage my calorie intake?

There are two different approaches to managing an 800 calorie intake on your fast days depending on your personal preferences and lifestyle.

- **OPTION 1: Skip breakfast, eat lunch & dinner.**
- **OPTION 2: Skip lunch, eat breakfast and dinner.**

There is much research and debate about the health benefits and risks of skipping meals, however the beauty of the 5:2 Diet is that the fasting occurs only for 2 days of the week with the remaining 5 reserved for 'normal' eating and recommended daily calorie intakes (1900-2000 for women, 2400-2500 for men). This means there is not a prolonged period of starving the body of calories, and eating balanced meals like those included in this book ensures that nutrition is still provided on the fasting days.

Our recipes are divided into breakfast, lunch and dinner. You choose meals from any chapter as long as they stay under a total of 800 calories when the calories are combined. Remember that drinks during the day such as tea and coffee will also count towards your calorie limit so remember to account for these. You can also make some meals more substantial if you need to increase calories by adding side dishes (see the suggestions at the end of this introduction).

portion sizes

The size of the portion that you put on your plate will significantly affect your weight loss efforts. Filling your plate with over-sized portions will obviously increase your calorie intake and hamper your dieting efforts.

It's important that with all meals, both on your fasting and normal eating days, you use a correct sized portion, which generally is the size of your clenched fist. This applies to any side dishes of vegetables and carbs too. You will be surprised at how quickly you will adopt this as the 'norm' as the weeks go by and you will begin to stop over-eating.

measurements

Most of our recipes serve 4 meaning you can either cook for a family or portion and divide for another day making it easy to pre-plan your fast day menu. As with portion sizes, stick with the recommended measurements of ingredients. Altering these will affect your calorie intake and therefore your ultimate weight loss.

choosing your fast days

Give yourself the best possible chance of success by choosing your fast days in advance and sticking to them. As we have already said, we recommend choosing two non-consecutive fasting days so that you only have one 24-hour period at a time where you have to concentrate on limiting your calories.

It makes sense to choose your fast days sensibly based on your own particular lifestyle. For example, for many, a Friday night may involve takeaway food after a hard week at work. If this is your ritual, then avoid this as your fasting day. Similarly if you meet up with friends during the week or have a business event that is likely to involve lunch or dinner then choose an alternative day. You can alter the days each week but just remember to check your calendars and prepare in advance.

nutrition

All of the recipes in this collection are balanced low calorie meals which should keep you feeling full on your fasting days.

In any diet, it is important to balance your food between proteins, good carbs, dairy, fruit and vegetables.

●   Protein. Keeps you feeling full and is also essential for building body tissue. Good protein sources come from meat, fish and eggs.
●   Carbohydrates. Not all carbs are good and generally they are high in calories which makes them difficult to include in a calorie limiting diet. Carbs are a good source of energy for your body as they are converted more easily into glucose (sugar) providing energy. Try to eat 'good carbs' which are high in fibre and nutrients e.g. whole fruits and veg, nuts, seeds, whole grain cereals, beans and legumes.
●   Dairy. Dairy products provide you with vitamins and minerals. Cheeses can be very high in calories. Other products such as low fat Greek yoghurt, crème fraiche and skimmed milk are all good.
●   Fruit & Vegetables. Eat your five a day. There is never a better time to fill your 5 a day quota. Not only are fruit and veg very healthy, they also fill up your plate and are ideal snacks when you are feeling hungry.

some fasting tips

●   Avoid too much exercise on your fasting days. Eating less is likely to make you feel a little weaker, certainly to start with, so don't put the pressure on yourself to exercise.

- Avoid alcohol on your fasting days. Not only is alcohol packed with calories, it could also have a greater effect on you than usual as you haven't eaten as much.
- Don't give up! Even if you find your fasting days tough to start with, stick with it. Remember you can eat what you like tomorrow without having to feel guilty.
- Drink plenty of water throughout the day. Water is the best friend you have on your fasting days. It's good for you, has zero calories, and will fill you up and help stop you feeling hungry.
- When you are eating each meal, put your fork down between bites – it will make you eat more slowly and you'll feel fuller on less food.
- Drink a glass of water before and also with your meal. Again this will help you feel fuller.
- Brush your teeth immediately after your meal to discourage yourself from eating more.
- Have clear motivations. Think about what you are trying to achieve and stick with it. Remember you can eat what you want tomorrow.
- If unwanted food cravings do strike, acknowledge them, then distract yourself. Go out for a walk, phone a friend, play with the kids, or paint your nails.
- Whenever hunger hits, try waiting 15 minutes and ride out the cravings. You'll find they pass and you can move on with your day.
- Remember - feeling hungry is not a bad thing. We are all so used to acting on the smallest hunger pangs that we forget what it's like to feel genuinely hungry. Feeling hungry for a couple of days a week is not going to harm you. Learn to 'own' your hunger and take control of how you deal with it.
- If you feel you can't do it by yourself then get some support. Encourage a friend or partner to join you on the 5:2 Diet. Having someone to talk things through with can be a real help.
- Get moving. Being active isn't a necessity for fasting to have results but as with all diets increased activity will complement your weight loss efforts. Think about what you are doing each day: choose the stairs instead of the lift, walk to the shops instead of driving. Making small changes will not only help you burn calories but will make you feel healthier and more in control of your weight loss.
- Don't beat yourself up! If you have a bad day forget about it, don't feel guilty. Recognise where you went wrong and move on. Tomorrow is a new day and you can start all over again. Fast for just two days a week and you'll see results. Guaranteed!

calorie conscious side suggestions

If you want to make any of the recipes or snacks in this book more substantial you may want to add an accompaniment to them. Here's a list of some key side vegetables, salad, noodles etc which you may find useful when working out your calories.

All calories are per 100g/3½ oz. Rice and noodle measurements are cooked weights.

- Asparagus: 20 cals
- Beansprouts: 30 cals
- Brussel Sprouts: 42 cals
- Butternut Squash: 45 cals
- Cabbage: 30 cals

- Carrots: 41 cals
- Cauliflower: 25 cals
- Celery: 14 cals
- Courgette/zucchini: 16 cals
- Cucumber: 15 cals
- Egg noodles: 62 cals
- Green beans: 81 cals
- Leeks: 61 cals
- Long grain rice: 140 cals
- Mixed salad leaves: 17 cals
- Mushrooms: 22 cals
- Pak choi; 13 cals
- Parsnips: 67 cals
- Peas: 64 cals

- Pepper (bell): 20 cals
- Potatoes: 75 cals
- Rocket: 17 cals
- Shirataki 'Miracle' noodles: 30 cals
- Spinach: 23 cals
- Sweet Potato: 86 cals
- Sweet corn: 86 cals
- Tomatoes: 18 cals

RAPID

800

BREAKFAST

balsamic garlic & rosemary tomatoes

- 12 large beef tomatoes, quartered
- 4 garlic cloves, crushed
- 2 tsp dried rosemary
- 2 tbsp olive oil
- 1 tbsp balsamic vinegar
- 2 onions, sliced
- 2 small ciabatta rolls
- Salt & pepper to taste

240 calories

- Combine together the crushed garlic, rosemary, olive oil & balsamic vinegar and gently heat in a frying pan.

- Season the tomatoes and saute in the frying pan along with the onions for 8-10 minutes or until the tomatoes are softened and cooked through.

- Cut the ciabatta rolls in half and lightly toast. Pile the balsamic onions and tomatoes on top of the ciabatta halves and serve.

Red onions and plum tomatoes make a great alternative.

mustard mushrooms on granary

- 1 tbsp olive oil
- 2 garlic cloves, crushed
- 1 onion, sliced
- 500g/1lb 2oz mushrooms, sliced
- 1 tbsp Dijon mustard
- 120ml/½ cup low fat crème fraiche

- 4 pieces granary bread, lightly toasted
- 2 tbsp freshly chopped flat leaf parsley
- Salt & pepper to taste

205 calories

- Gently saute the onions and garlic in the olive oil for a few minutes.

- Add the mushrooms and continue cooking for 8-10 minutes or until the mushrooms are soft and cooked through.

- Stir through the mustard and creme fraiche, combine well and warm through.

- Pile the creamy mushrooms and onions onto the granary toast and sprinkle with chopped parsley.

- Season and serve.

You could substitute English mustard in this recipe but it will be a lot 'hotter'!

cajun spinach eggs

- 2 red peppers, deseeded & sliced
- 1 tsp paprika
- ½ tsp each chilli powder, cumin, coriander & salt

- 8 large free-range eggs
- 1 tbsp olive oil
- 125g/4oz spinach leaves
- Salt & pepper to taste

210 calories

- Break the eggs into a bowl, add the dried spices & salt and lightly beat with a fork.

- Gently heat the oil in a frying pan and add the peppers.

- Saute for a few minutes until they begin to soften.

- Add the spinach and allow to wilt for a minute or two.

- Pour in the beaten eggs and move around the pan until the eggs begin to scramble. As soon as they start to set remove from the heat and serve with lots of black pepper.

You can use a ready made Cajun mix if you have one to hand.

berry smoothie

- 200g/7oz blueberries
- 300g/11oz strawberries
- 2 large ripe bananas

- 500ml/2 cups fat free Greek yogurt
- 2 tsp runny honey
- Lots of ice cubes

190 calories

- Remove the strawberry stalks and peel the bananas.

- Blend all the ingredients together.

- Check the sweetness of the smoothie and add a little more honey if needed.

- Divide into 4 glasses and serve immediately.

Add some Brazil nuts to the recipe when you blend for a slightly different texture.

blue cheese omelette

- 2 large free-range eggs
- 40g/1½oz stilton cheese, crumbled
- 1 tsp olive oil
- 50g/2oz watercress
- Salt & pepper to taste

330 calories

- Lightly beat the eggs with a fork. Season well and add the crumbled blue cheese.

- Gently heat the oil in a small frying pan and add the omelette mixture. Tilt the pan to ensure the mixture is evenly spread over the base.

- Cook on a low to medium heat and, when the eggs are set underneath, fold the omelette in half and continue to cook for a further 2 minutes.

- Serve with the watercress sprinkled all over the top.

Check the eggs are set underneath by lifting with a fork before folding the omelette in half.

mango & avocado breakfast salad

- 2 ripe avocados, peeled, stoned & cubed
- 1 ripe mango, peeled, stoned & cubed
- 250g/9oz plum tomatoes, diced
- ½ tsp paprika
- ½ red chilli, deseeded & finely chopped
- 1 red onion, finely chopped
- 2 tbsp lime juice
- 1 tbsp freshly chopped coriander
- 150g/5oz watercress or rocket leaves
- Salt & pepper to taste

140 calories

- Combine the cubed avocado, mango, tomatoes, paprika, onions, chilli, lime & coriander together.

- Put to one side and allow to sit for a few minutes to let the flavour infuse.

- Pile onto a bed of watercress or rocket leaves, season & serve.

Stone the avocados by cutting in half. Use a knife to lever out the stone then scoop each half out in one piece.

scrambled vegetable omelette

- 400g/14oz baby new potatoes, halved
- 125g/4oz tenderstem broccoli, roughly chopped
- 1 tbsp olive oil
- 1 onion, sliced
- 1 tsp turmeric & paprika
- ½ tsp chilli powder
- 8 large free-range eggs
- Salt & pepper to taste

260 calories

- Place the potatoes and chopped broccoli in salted boiling water. Boil for 4-6 minutes or until the potatoes are tender. Drain and put to one side.

- Meanwhile gently heat the olive oil in a frying pan and saute the onions for a few minutes until softened.

- Add the potatoes, broccoli & dried spices to the pan and stir. Cook for a minute or two longer before adding the eggs to the pan.

- Increase the heat and cook until the eggs are scrambled. Check the seasoning & serve immediately.

Try this recipe substituting the turmeric for ground coriander and garnishing with fresh chopped coriander leaves.

parmesan & roasted pepper frittata

- 1 tbsp olive oil
- 1 onion, chopped
- 125g/4oz courgettes, sliced
- 250g/9oz roasted peppers, drained & chopped
- 10 free-range eggs

- 1 tbsp grated Parmesan cheese
- 2 tbsp freshly chopped flat leaf parsley
- Salt & pepper to taste
-

246 calories

- Heat the oil in a frying pan and gently saute the onions and courgettes for a few minutes until softened.

- Add the peppers and continue to cook for 2-3 minutes longer.

- Break the eggs into a bowl and combine with Parmesan cheese. Tip the softened onions and courgettes into the bowl. Mix well and return the eggs & vegetables to the pan, tilting to ensure the mixture covers the base evenly.

- Cover the pan, reduce the heat and leave to cook for a few minutes. Flip the frittata over and cook the other side until the eggs set and the vegetables are tender.

- Cut into wedges and serve with chopped parsley sprinkled over the top.

To keep things really simple use jars of pre-cooked roasted peppers for this recipe.

victorian breakfast

- 8 fresh lambs' kidneys
- 1 tbsp olive oil
- 4 garlic cloves, crushed
- 75g/3oz button mushrooms, halved
- 1 onion, sliced
- 2 tbsp Worcestershire sauce

- 1 tsp cayenne pepper
- 120ml/½ cup low fat crème fraiche
- 75g/3oz spinach leaves
- 2 English breakfast muffins, lightly toasted
- Salt & pepper to taste

330 calories

- Prepare the lambs' kidneys by cutting in half and trimming out any tough core.

- Gently saute the garlic, mushrooms & onions for a few minutes until softened.

- Add the kidneys, Worcestershire sauce and cayenne pepper to the pan. Combine well and cook the kidneys for approx. 4-5 minutes each side.

- When the kidneys are cooked through, stir in the creme fraiche and spinach and warm through.

- Season and serve on the toasted English muffins.

Lambs' kidneys are a traditional breakfast often served during the Victorian era - the spinach is a contemporary addition!

eggs & mushrooms

- 8 tsp low fat soft cheese
- 2 tbsp freshly chopped chives
- 2 garlic cloves, crushed
- 8 large flat mushrooms

- 4 large free-range eggs
- 1 handful rocket leaves
- Salt & pepper to taste

140 calories

- Preheat the oven grill.

- Mix the soft cheese, chives & garlic together and spread evenly on the underside of each mushroom.

- Season well and place, underside up, under the grill for 6-10 minutes or until the mushrooms are cooked through.

- Meanwhile fill a frying pan with boiling water and break the eggs into the gently simmering pan to poach while the mushrooms cook.

- Put the mushrooms on the plates. Arrange the rocket over the top and add a poached egg.

- Serve with lots of black pepper.

You can buy low fat soft cheese with chives already added.

scrambled truffle eggs

- 1 tsp butter
- 50g/2oz shallots, chopped
- Pinch of chilli flakes
- 1 tsp truffle oil
- 2 medium free-range eggs

- 1 tbsp freshly chopped flat leaf parsley
- 50g/2oz rocket
- Salt & pepper to taste

240 calories

- Gently heat the butter in a frying pan and sauté the chopped shallots and chilli flakes for a few minutes until the shallots are softened.

- Add the eggs to the pan. Increase the heat. Keep moving everything quickly around the pan and cook until the eggs are scrambled.

- Check the seasoning and serve with the rocket piled on the side of the plate.

- Drizzle the truffle oil over the top and sprinkle with chopped parsely.

Truffle oil gives this breakfast a luxurious finish.

RAPID

800

LUNCH

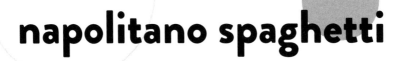

napolitano spaghetti

- 300g/11oz dried spaghetti
- 2 tbsp olive oil
- 400g/14oz cherry tomatoes, roughly chopped
- 200g/7oz pitted black olives, roughly chopped
- 2 stalks celery, finely chopped
- 1 onion, finely chopped
- 3 garlic cloves, crushed
- 1 tbsp tomato puree
- 4 tbsp freshly chopped basil
- Salt & pepper to taste

410 calories

- Heat the oil and gently saute the tomatoes, olives, celery, onions, garlic, tomato puree & basil for 10-15 minutes or until the tomatoes lose their shape and combine to make a sauce.

- Whilst the sauce is cooking place the spaghetti in a pan of salted boiling water until tender. Drain the cooked pasta and add to the frying pan.

- Toss well, season & serve.

You could cook the sauce for much longer if you have the time to increase the richness of the dish.

flaked salmon fillet & savoy cabbage

- 500g/1lb 2oz skinless salmon fillets
- 1 Savoy cabbage, shredded
- 1 tbsp olive oil
- 2 garlic cloves, crushed

- 2 tbsp freshly chopped chives
- 2 tbsp low fat crème fraiche
- 2 tbsp horseradish sauce
- 2 tbsp lemon juice
- Salt & pepper to taste

329 calories

● Season the salmon fillets and place under a preheated grill for 10-12 minutes or until cooked through. Flake and put to one side to cool.

● Steam the cabbage for 8-10 minutes or until the cabbage is tender.

● Meanwhile heat the oil and garlic in a saucepan and gently saute for a minute or two. Add the cooked cabbage, stir well and cook for a minute or two longer.

● Gently combine together the chives, creme fraiche, horseradish sauce, lemon juice & flaked salmon.

● Divide the dressed salmon and sauteed cabbage onto plates, season & serve.

Feel free to use pre-cooked salmon fillets if you are short of time.

dolcelatte chicken salad

- 500g/1lb 2oz skinless chicken breast
- 200g/7oz cherry tomatoes
- 100g/3½oz Dolcelatte cheese
- 2 ripe avocados, peeled & stoned

- 2 tbsp extra virgin olive oil
- 2 tbsp cider vinegar
- 2 tbsp low fat crème fraiche
- 1 tsp paprika
- 200g/7oz watercress
- Salt & pepper to taste

520 calories

- Season the chicken fillets and place under a preheated grill for 15-20 minutes or until cooked through. Slice into strips and put to one side to cool.

- Halve the cherry tomatoes and crumble the Dolcelatte cheese.

- Combine together the olive oil, vinegar, creme fraiche & paprika to make a dressing.

- Toss the dressing, tomatoes, cheese, avocados & watercress together in a large bowl.

- Divide onto plates and arrange the chicken slices on top. Season and serve.

Feta cheese also works well in this recipe.

veggie couscous

- 1 tbsp olive oil
- 2 courgettes, sliced
- 2 red peppers, deseeded & sliced
- 2 tbsp pitted black olives, chopped
- 1 onion, chopped
- 2 garlic cloves, crushed
- 1 tsp ground coriander

- 1 tbsp lemon juice
- 1½/370ml cups vegetable stock
- 200g/7oz couscous
- 2 tbsp sultanas, chopped
- Lemon wedges to serve
- 2 tbsp freshly chopped coriander
- Salt & pepper to taste

- Gently saute the courgettes, peppers, olives, onions, garlic, ground coriander & lemon juice for a 7-10 minutes or until softened and cooked through.

- Whilst the vegetables are cooking, place the couscous & sultanas is a pan with the hot stock.

- Bring the pan to the boil, remove from the heat, cover and leave to stand for 3-4 minutes or until all the stock is absorbed and the couscous is tender.

- Fluff the couscous with a fork and pile into the pan with the cooked vegetables. Mix well, divide onto plates and serve with fresh lemon wedges on the side & chopped coriander sprinkled over the top.

This is good served with a rocket or watercress salad.

anchovy & garlic spaghettini

- 300g/11oz dried spaghettini
- 12 tinned anchovy fillets, drained
- 4 tbsp olive oil
- 4 garlic cloves, crushed
- 2 red onions, sliced
- 3 tbsp lemon juice
- 4 tbsp freshly chopped basil
- Salt & pepper to taste

410 calories

- Cook the pasta in a pan of salted boiling water until tender.

- Place the anchovy fillets and oil in a high-sided frying pan and gently saute along with the garlic, red onions & lemon juice whilst the pasta cooks. After a little while the anchovy fillets should dissolve to make a salty sauce base.

- When the pasta is tender, drain and add to the frying pan.

- Combine really well to make sure every strand spaghettini is covered with the oil and anchovy sauce.

- Sprinkle with the freshly chopped basil. Season & serve.

If the tinned anchovies are stored in olive oil, reserve the drained fishy oil and use to cook the onions instead of plain kitchen olive oil.

fresh pea & prawn noodles

- 1 tbsp olive oil
- 4 garlic cloves, crushed
- 1 tbsp freshly grated ginger
- ½ tsp crushed chilli flakes
- 500g/1lb 2oz shelled, raw king prawns
- 1 onion, sliced
- 60ml/¼ cup soy sauce
- 2 red peppers, deseeded & sliced
- 2 tbsp Thai fish sauce
- 200g/7oz fresh peas
- 400g/14oz straight to wok noodles
- Lemon wedges to serve
- Salt & pepper to taste

350 calories

- Heat the olive oil in a frying pan and gently saute the garlic and ginger for a minute.

- Add the chilli flakes, prawns, onions, peppers, soy sauce, fish sauce & fresh peas and cook for 8-10 minutes or until the peppers soften and the prawns pink up.

- Add the noodles and combine for 3-4 minutes or until the noodles are piping hot and the prawns are cooked through.

- Season and serve with lemon wedges.

This simple stir-fry works equally well with sliced chicken breast.

33

broccoli & chicken stir-fry

- 400g/14oz skinless chicken breast, sliced
- 400g/14oz tenderstem broccoli
- 1 tbsp olive oil
- 2 garlic cloves, crushed
- 1 onion, chopped

- 2 tbsp soy sauce
- 60ml/¼ cup chicken stock
- 200g/7oz spinach leaves, chopped
- 250g/9oz rice
- Salt & pepper to taste

420 calories

- Season the chicken and roughly chop the broccoli.

- Place the rice in salted boiling water and cook until tender.

- Meanwhile heat the olive oil in a frying pan and gently saute the garlic and onions for a few minutes.

- Add the chicken & chopped broccoli to the pan along with the soy sauce and chicken stock.

- Stir-fry for 8-10 minutes until the chicken is cooked through.

- Add the drained rice to the pan along with the spinach.

- Combine for a minute or two, check the seasoning and serve.

As a time saver microwaveable rice is a handy store cupboard ingredient for super fast stir-frys.

coriander chicken & rice

SERVES 4

- 250g/9oz rice
- 2 tbsp coriander seeds
- 2 tbsp fenugreek seeds
- 1 tbsp olive oil
- 2 garlic cloves, crushed
- 2 tbsp soy sauce
- 1 red chilli, deseeded & finely chopped
- 400g/14oz skinless chicken breast, sliced
- 2 large free-range eggs
- Salt & pepper to taste

510 calories

- Place the rice in salted boiling water and cook until tender.

- Meanwhile bash the coriander and fenugreek seeds with a pestle and mortar.

- Heat the olive oil in a frying pan and gently saute the garlic for a minute along with the bashed seeds.

- Add the chilli, chicken & soy sauce and cook for 5-10 minutes or until the chicken is cooked through.

- Add the drained rice to the pan along with the eggs. Increase the heat, stir-fry for 3-4 minutes.

- Season & serve.

Freshly chopped coriander makes a good garnish for this dish.

chinese pak choi & prawns

- 250g/9oz rice
- 2 pak choi
- 60ml/¼ cup chicken stock
- 1 tbsp olive oil
- 2 garlic cloves, crushed
- 1 onion, sliced
- 1 tbsp freshly grated ginger

- 500g/1lb 2oz shelled raw king prawns
- 1 tbsp soy sauce
- 2 tsp Chinese five spice powder
- 1 tsp crushed chilli flakes
- Salt & pepper to taste

365 calories

- Place the rice in salted boiling water and cook until tender.

- Shred the pak choi and gently wilt in a frying pan with the chicken stock for a few minutes until tender.

- Heat the olive oil in a frying pan and saute the garlic, onions & ginger for a minute or two.

- Add the prawns, soy sauce, Chinese five spice powder & chilli flakes and cook until the prawns are pink. Check the prawns are cooked through.

- Add the drained rice to the pan and combine for a minute or two.

- Quickly toss through the pak choi. Season and serve immediately.

Pak choi is a widely available oriental cabbage but any type of cabbage will work well.

peppers & steak

SERVES 4

- 400g/14oz sirloin steak
- 2 tbsp olive oil
- 1 tsp paprika
- 1 onion, sliced
- 2 garlic cloves, crushed
- 4 red & yellow peppers, deseeded & sliced

- 400g/14oz cherry tomatoes
- 4 baby gem lettuces, shredded
- 50g/2oz feta cheese, crumbled
- Salt & pepper to taste

420 calories

- Trim any fat off the steak. Lightly brush with a little of the olive oil & all the paprika. Season and put a frying pan on a high heat.

- In another pan gently saute the peppers, onions & garlic in the rest of the olive oil for 5-7 minutes or until tender.

- Place the steak in the smoking hot dry pan and cook for 1-2 minutes each side, or to your liking. Leave to rest for 3 minutes and then finely slice.

- Halve the tomatoes & shred the lettuces. Add the peppers, crumble the feta cheese and combine on plates.

- Place the sliced steak on top. Season and serve.

You could choose to use Stilton cheese instead of feta for this lovely fresh recipe.

tuna steak & spiced courgettes

- 300g/11oz courgettes, diced
- 1 red onion, finely chopped
- 2 tbsp olive oil
- 6 tbsp balsamic vinegar

- 4 fresh tuna steaks, each weighing 125g/4oz
- 400g/14oz watercress
- Salt & pepper to taste

270 calories

- Gently saute the courgettes and red onion in 1 tbsp of olive oil for a few minutes until softened.

- Season the tuna and put a frying pan on a high heat with the rest of the olive oil and balsamic vinegar.

- Place the tuna in the pan and cook for 2 minutes each side.

- Remove the tuna from the pan and serve with the watercress and courgette side dish.

Two minutes of cooking each side should leave the tuna rare in the centre. Reduce or increase cooking time depending on your preference.

oregano & chilli spaghetti

- 300g/11oz dried spaghetti
- 2 tsp dried oregano
- ½ tsp crushed chilli flakes
- 2 tbsp pitted black olives, chopped
- 1 onion, sliced
- 4 tbsp sundried tomato puree
- 2 tbsp olive oil
- Salt & pepper to taste

350 calories

● Cook the spaghetti in a pan of salted boiling water until tender.

● Meanwhile gently saute the oregano, chilli, olives, onions & sundried tomato puree for a few minutes or until the onions are softened.

● Drain the cooked pasta and add to the pan.

● Toss well, season & serve.

If you don't have sundried tomato puree, you could use chopped sundried tomatoes and regular tomato puree.

porcini & thyme linguine

SERVES 4

- 50g/2oz dried porcini mushrooms
- 300g/11oz dried linguine
- 1 tbsp olive oil
- 2 garlic cloves, crushed
- 1 onion, sliced

- 2 tsp dried thyme
- 2 tbsp low fat mascarpone cheese
- 1 tbsp tomato puree
- Salt & pepper to taste

370 calories

- Place the porcini mushrooms in a little boiling water and leave to rehydrate for 10-15 minutes. Thinly slice when softened.

- Cook the spaghetti in a pan of salted boiling water until tender.

- Heat the olive oil in a high-sided frying pan and gently saute the garlic, onions & dried thyme whilst the pasta cooks.

- When the onions are soft add the mascarpone cheese, and tomato puree and stir well. Drain the cooked pasta and add to the frying pan.

- Toss well. Season & serve.

Dried porcini mushrooms are readily available in any supermarket.

prawn & chorizo angel hair pasta

- 300g/11oz dried angel hair pasta
- 1 tbsp olive oil
- 2 garlic cloves, crushed
- 50g/2oz chorizo, finely chopped or sliced
- 1 tsp paprika
- 1 onion, sliced
- 250g/9oz shelled raw king prawns, chopped
- 4 tbsp lemon juice
- 4 tsp freshly chopped flat leaf parsley
- Salt & pepper to taste

420 calories

- Cook the spaghetti in a pan of salted boiling water until tender.

- Meanwhile heat the olive oil in a high-sided frying pan and gently saute the garlic, chorizo, paprika and onions for 5 minutes whilst the pasta cooks.

- Add the chopped prawns and lemon juice and cook until the prawns are pink and cooked through.

- Drain the cooked pasta, add to the frying pan and combine really well.

- Sprinkle with chopped parsley and serve.

Chorizo and shellfish are a classic combination. Serve with lots of freshly ground black pepper.

cod, asparagus & avocado

- 2 garlic cloves, crushed
- 2 tbsp olive oil
- 200g/7oz asparagus spears
- 4 boneless, skinless cod fillets each weighing 125g/4oz
- 250g/9oz ripe plum tomatoes, finely chopped
- 2 avocados, peeled & stoned

- 1 bunch spring onions, finely chopped
- 2 tbsp freshly chopped oregano
- 200g/7oz watercress
- 1 lime, cut into wedges
- Salt & pepper to taste
-

315 calories

- Mix together the garlic & olive oil and brush onto the cod fillets & asparagus spears.

- Place the fish and asparagus under a preheated grill and cook for 5-7 minutes or until the cod is cooked through and the asparagus spears are tender

- Meanwhile combine the chopped tomatoes, spring onions, avocados, chopped oregano & watercress together.

- Season and serve the cooked cod with the watercress tomato salad & lime wedges.

Any firm white fish will work just as well for this dish.

pan fried lemon & paprika haddock

- 4 boneless, skinless haddock fillets each weighing 125g/4oz
- 1 onion, sliced
- 200g/7oz mushrooms
- 1 tsp each paprika & mixed spice

- 3 tbsp lemon juice
- 2 tbsp olive oil
- 150g/5oz rocket
- Salt & pepper to taste

190 calories

- Season the haddock fillets.

- Gently saute the garlic in the olive oil for a few minutes.

- Add the onions, mushrooms, paprika, mixed spice & lemon juice and cook for 5-8 minutes or until the onions are softened.

- Move the vegetables to one side of the pan to make room for the haddock fillets. Cook for 3-5 minutes each side depending on the thickness of the fillet, or until cooked through.

- Serve the cooked haddock fillets on a bed of rocket with the onions & mushrooms arranged over the top of the fish.

Serve with lemon wedges and chopped parsley if you wish.

creamy leek & potato soup

- 500g/1lb 2oz potatoes
- 500g/1lb 2oz leeks
- 1lt/4 cups vegetable stock/broth
- 60ml/¼ cup low fat single cream
- Salt & pepper to taste

150 calories

- Peel and chop the potatoes & leeks.

- Place the potatoes and leeks in a saucepan with the hot stock.

- Bring to the boil and leave to simmer for 10-12 minutes or until the potatoes and tender.

- Blend the soup to a smooth consistency, stir through the cream, check the seasoning and serve.

Add some freshly chopped herbs to garnish if you wish.

horseradish mackerel & spinach

- 4 fresh, boned headless mackerel each weighing 150g/5oz
- 1 tsp turmeric
- 2 tsp curry powder
- 1 tbsp olive oil

- 2 tbsp horseradish sauce
- 1 tbsp lemon juice
- 2 tbsp chopped capers
- 300g/11oz spinach
- Salt & pepper to taste

350 calories

- Butterfly each mackerel to open into one large flat fillet. Season each fish and rub with turmeric and curry powder.

- Heat the olive oil in a pan and fry the mackerel for 3 minutes each side.

- Meanwhile combine together the horseradish sauce, lemon juice & capers to make a dressing.

- When the fish is cooked, wrap in foil and put to one side to keep warm.

- Add the spinach to the empty pan and cook for a few minutes. Stir the dressing through the wilted spinach and serve with the cooked mackerel fillets.

Use shop-bought horseradish or make your own by combining freshly grated horseradish, crème fraiche, lemon juice & Dijon mustard.

broccoli & cauliflower soup

- 200g/7oz cauliflower florets, chopped
- 200g/7oz broccoli florets, chopped
- 75g/3oz potatoes, peeled & chopped
- 1 onion, chopped

- 1 tsp ground coriander
- 1lt/4 cups vegetable stock/ broth
- 250ml/1 cup semi skimmed milk
- Salt & pepper to taste

90 calories

- Add all the ingredients, except the milk, to the saucepan.

- Bring to the boil and leave to simmer for 10-12 minutes or until the vegetables are tender.

- Blend to a smooth consistency, add the milk, and heat through for a minute or two.

- Check the seasoning and serve.

Freshly chopped chives or flat leaf parsley make a lovely garnish for this soup.

chilli prawns & mango

- 250g/9oz rice
- 1 red pepper, deseeded & sliced
- 1 onion, sliced
- 2 garlic cloves, crushed
- 1 tbsp freshly grated ginger
- ½ tsp brown sugar
- 1 tbsp olive oil
- 1 tbsp soy sauce
- 1 tsp dried chilli flakes

- 500g/1lb 2oz shelled raw king prawns
- 1 mango, stoned & finely chopped
- 4 tbsp freshly chopped coriander
- 2 tbsp lime juice
- Salt & pepper

395 calories

● Place the rice in salted boiling water and cook until tender.

● Gently saute the sliced peppers, onions, garlic, ginger & sugar in the olive oil for a few minutes until softened.

● Add the prawns & chilli flakes and cook for 5-8 minutes or until the prawns are pink and cooked through.

● Add the drained rice to the pan, combine well and cook together for a minute or two longer.

● Combine together the mango, coriander and lime juice to make a mango salsa.

● Divide the prawns and rice into bowls and serve with the mango salsa piled on top.

Reduce the amount of crushed chillies in the dish if you don't want the meal to have too much 'kick'.

parmesan crusted salmon

- 500g/1lb 2oz baby new potatoes, halved
- 4 boneless, skinless salmon fillets each weighing 125g/4oz
- 2 tbsp grated Parmesan cheese
- 6 tbsp fresh breadcrumbs

- 2 garlic cloves, crushed
- 200g/7oz tenderstem broccoli
- Lemon wedges to serve
- Salt & pepper to taste

- Cook the new potatoes in a pan of salted boiling water until tender.

- Meanwhile season the salmon fillets. Mix the Parmesan cheese, breadcrumbs & garlic together and coat the top of the salmon fillets with the breadcrumb mixture.

- Place the salmon under a preheated grill and cook for 10-13 minutes or until the salmon fillets are cooked through.

- Whilst the salmon and potatoes are cooking plunge the broccoli into salted boiling water and cook for a 2-3 minutes or until tender.

- Drain the potatoes and broccoli and serve with the salmon fillets and lemon wedges.

To make fresh breadcrumbs place slices of bread in the food processor and pulse for a few seconds.

mushroom & caramelised onion soup

SERVES 4

- 1 tsp olive oil
- 2 garlic cloves, crushed
- 2 onions, chopped
- 2 tbsp balsamic vinegar
- 200g/7oz potatoes, peeled & diced
- 500g/1lb 2oz mushrooms, sliced
- 1ltml/4 cups vegetable stock/ broth
- Salt & pepper to taste

115 calories

- Heat the oil in a saucepan and add the garlic, onions & balsamic vinegar.

- Saute on a high heat until the onions are cooked crispy brown and the balsamic vinegar reduces down. Put to one side when caramelised.

- Meanwhile add the potatoes, mushrooms & stock to a saucepan. Bring to the boil and simmer for 8-10 minutes or until the potatoes are soft.

- Blend to a smooth consistency and divide into bowls.

- Split the onions equally and place in the centre of each bowl of soup. Season and serve.

Add some chopped chives if you like and serve with crusty bread!

chicken noodle ramen

- 2 leeks, sliced
- 2 celery stalks, chopped
- 2 carrots, chopped
- 1 tsp dried thyme
- 1lt/4 cups chicken stock
- 1 bunch spring onions, sliced thinly lengthways

- 250g/9oz cooked chicken breast, shredded
- 200g/7oz tinned sweetcorn, drained
- 400g/14oz straight to wok ramen noodles
- Salt & pepper to taste

330 calories

- Place the leeks, celery and carrots in a saucepan along with the thyme and stock.

- Bring to the boil and simmer for 7-10 minutes or until all the vegetables are soft.

- Blend to a smooth consistency and return to the pan.

- Add the shredded chicken, sweetcorn & noodles and cook for a further 4-6 minutes or until the ramen is piping hot.

- Check the seasoning and serve with the sliced spring onions on top.

Dried noodles are fine to use too. Just use half the quantity and cook for a little longer in the stock.

fresh asparagus & watercress soup

- 125g/4oz potatoes, finely chopped
- 1 tbsp olive oil
- 2 garlic cloves, crushed
- 1 tsp dried thyme
- 1 onion, sliced

- 750ml/3 cups vegetable stock/broth
- 400g/14oz asparagus tips
- 250ml/1 cup dry white wine
- 150g/5oz watercress
- Salt & pepper to taste

150 calories

- Add all the ingredients, except the watercress, to a saucepan.

- Bring to the boil and simmer for 5-7 minutes, or until the potatoes are tender.

- Roughly blend the soup with just a couple of pulses in the food processor.

- Stir through the watercress, check the seasoning and serve immediately.

You could use rocket or spinach rather than watercress if you wish.

lemon & basil zucchini gnocchi

SERVES 4

- 3 tbsp olive oil
- 2 garlic cloves, crushed
- 300g/11oz baby courgettes, thinly sliced lengthways
- 4 tbsp lemon juice
- 4 tbsp freshly chopped basil
- 700g/1lb 9oz gnocchi
- Salt & pepper to taste

355 calories

- Gently heat the olive oil in a frying pan and saute the garlic, courgettes, lemon juice & basil.

- Meanwhile place the gnocchi in a pan of salted boiling water.

- Cook for 2-3 minutes or until the gnocchi begins to float to the top.

- As soon as the gnocchi is cooked, drain and place in the frying pan with the courgettes on a high heat.

- Move the gnocchi around for a minute or two to coat each dumpling in oil. Season and serve.

Chopped spinach also makes a nice addition to this veggie dish.

penne, peas & beans

- 150g/5oz baby broad beans
- 300g/11oz dried penne
- 1 tbsp olive oil
- 2 garlic cloves, crushed
- 150g/5oz fresh peas
- 120ml/½ cup low fat crème fraiche
- 2 tbsp freshly chopped mint
- Salt & pepper to taste

380 calories

- Blanch the broad beans and remove the skins.

- Cook the penne in a pan of salted boiling water until tender.

- Meanwhile gently heat the olive oil in a high-sided frying pan and saute the blanched broad beans, garlic & peas whilst the pasta cooks.

- When the peas and beans are cooked through stir in the creme fraiche and mint.

- Drain the cooked penne and add to the pan.

- Toss well, season & serve with lots of freshly ground black pepper.

Blanch the beans by plunging in unsalted boiling water for 3-4 minutes. Drain, cover with cold water & slide off the skins.

warm cucumber tuna salad

- 1 cucumber, finely sliced into matchsticks
- 2 tsp caster sugar
- 120ml/½ cup rice wine vinegar
- ½ tsp dried chilli flakes
- 1 red onion, finely chopped
- 400g/14oz tinned tuna, drained
- 400g/14oz tinned borlotti beans, drained & rinsed
- 125g/4oz cherry tomatoes, halved
- 200g/7oz rocket
- Salt & pepper to taste

310 calories

- Place the cucumber in a frying pan and gently warm over a low heat.

- Add the caster sugar, rice wine vinegar & chilli flakes. Simmer for a few minutes and set aside to cool.

- Meanwhile mix together the red onion, beans, tomatoes & tuna in a large bowl.

- Add the cooled cucumber, toss with the rocket and serve.

This is a simple Asian salad. You may need to balance the sugar and vinegar a little.

avocado & prawn cocktail

- 2 tbsp low fat mayonnaise
- 2 tbsp low fat crème fraiche
- 2 tsp tomato ketchup
- 1 dash tobasco sauce
- 1 tbsp lemon juice
- 2 tbsp freshly chopped chives
- 500g/1lb 2oz cooked & peeled prawns

- 2 Romaine lettuces, shredded
- 2 ripe avocados, peeled, stoned & diced
- 1 cucumber, diced
- 1 tsp cayenne pepper
- Salt & pepper to taste
-

260 calories

- Mix together the mayonnaise, creme fraiche, ketchup, tobasco sauce, lemon juice, chives & prawns until everything is really well combined.

- In a separate bowl gently combine the shredded lettuce, avocado & cucumber to make a salad.

- Divide the salad on four plates and pile the dressed prawns on top

- Sprinkle with cayenne pepper and serve.

Use paprika rather than cayenne pepper if you want to reduce the 'heat'.

almond & onion sprout salad

- 500g/1lb 2oz prepared Brussels sprouts
- 3 tbsp olive oil
- 2 onions, sliced
- 150g/5oz blanched almonds
- Salt & pepper to taste

370
calories

- Slice the sprouts really thinly so they fall into shreds.

- Heat the olive oil in a frying pan and gently saute the onions for 8-10 minutes or until they are soft and golden.

- Meanwhile plunge the shredded sprouts into salted boiling water for 2 minutes.

- Drain and rinse through with cold water. Add to the onion pan along with the almonds and toss until piping hot and cooked through.

- Season with plenty of salt & freshly ground pepper to serve.

To blanch almonds: place the almonds in a bowl of boiling water for one minute. Drain & rinse under cold water. Pat dry and slip off their skins.

prawn & paprika rice

- 1 tbsp olive oil
- 2 garlic cloves, crushed
- 1 onion, sliced
- 2 red peppers, deseeded & sliced
- 1 tbsp paprika

- 300g/11oz cherry tomatoes, halved
- 250g/9oz rice
- 400g/14oz peeled raw prawns
- Salt & pepper to taste

380 calories

● Heat the olive oil in a frying pan and gently saute the garlic, onions, peppers & tomatoes for 15-20 minutes or until everything is softened and forms a combined base.

● Meanwhile place the rice in salted boiling water and cook until tender.

● Add the prawns & paprika to the frying pan and cook until piping hot and cooked through.

● When the rice is ready, drain and add to the pan.

● Toss well. Season and serve.

Add a dash of water to the pan during cooking if it needs loosening up.

fresh salad broth

- 1 tbsp olive oil
- 1 garlic clove, crushed
- 1 onion, sliced
- 1 carrot, diced
- 150g/5oz potatoes, peeled & diced
- 2 tsp dried mixed herbs
- 1lt/4 cups chicken or vegetable stock
- 150g/5oz watercress, roughly chopped
- Salt & pepper to taste

95 calories

- Heat the olive oil in a pan and gently saute the garlic, sliced onions, carrots, potatoes & dried herbs for a few minutes until softened.

- Add the stock, bring to the boil, cover and leave to simmer for 10-15 minutes or until everything is tender.

- Blend to your preferred consistency and add the watercress.

- Stir through, season and serve immediately.

Any mix of dried herbs will work well with this light summery soup.

asparagus & portabella open sandwich

- 2 tbsp olive oil
- 20 asparagus spears, chopped
- 4 large portabella mushrooms, sliced
- 1 onion, sliced
- 1 tsp dried basil
- 3 tbsp lemon juice
- ½ tsp crushed chilli flakes
- 2 tbsp freshly chopped flat leaf parsley
- 2 ciabatta rolls
- Salt & pepper to taste

215 calories

● Heat the olive oil in a pan and gently saute the asparagus, mushrooms, onions & basil for a few minutes until softened.

● Meanwhile spilt the ciabatta rolls in half and gently toast.

● When the mushrooms and asparagus are tender add the lemon juice and chilli flakes.

● Stir through, season and serve on top of each ciabatta half with the chopped parsley sprinkled on top.

Don't overcook the asparagus, you don't want it to be too soft.

sicilian caponata

- 1 tbsp olive oil
- 2 aubergines, cubed
- 200g/7oz baby courgettes, sliced in half lengthways
- 1 tsp dried oregano
- 2 onions, sliced
- 1 celery stalk, chopped
- 2 garlic cloves, crushed
- 3 tbsp balsamic vinegar
- 1 tbsp capers, chopped
- 200g/7oz ripe plum tomatoes, roughly chopped
- 2 tbsp pitted black olives, sliced
- 2 tbsp sultanas, roughly chopped
- 200g/7oz rice
- Salt & pepper to taste

320 calories

- Gently saute the aubergines, courgettes, oregano, onions, celery and garlic in the olive oil for a few minutes until softened.

- Add the balsamic vinegar, capers, tomatoes, olives & sultanas and continue to cook for 20-25 minutes or until everything is cooked through and tender.

- Whilst the aubergines are cooking place the rice in salted boiling water and cook until tender.

- Add the drained rice to the pan. Combine well, season & serve.

Caponata is a southern Italian dish which can also be served cold!

RAPID
800
DINNER

steak & stilton sauce

- 500g/1lb 2oz sweet potatoes
- 4 sirloin steaks each weighing 125g/4oz
- 1 tbsp olive oil
- 200g/7oz fresh peas

- 75g/3oz stilton cheese
- 3 tbsp crème fraiche
- 120ml/½ cup chicken stock
- Salt & pepper to taste

500 calories

- Peel the sweet potatoes, cut into 1cm slices and cook in the saucepan for 10-12 minutes or until they are tender.

- Meanwhile trim any fat off the steak. Season and brush with the olive oil while you put a frying pan on a high heat.

- Place the steak in the smoking hot dry pan and cook for 1-2 minutes each side, or to your liking. When the steak is cooked put to one side to rest for 3 minutes.

- Whilst the steak is resting quickly cook the peas in salted boiling water for a minute or two. In a separate pan gently heat and stir the stilton, creme fraiche and stock to make a sauce.

- Serve the steak, sweet potatoes & fresh peas with the stilton sauce drizzled over the top.

Adjust the steak cooking time depending on your preference and the thickness of the cut.

chicken, raisins & rice

- 250g/9oz rice
- 1 tbsp olive oil
- 3 garlic cloves, crushed
- 1 onion, chopped
- 200g/7oz raisins
- 500g/1lb 2oz skinless chicken breast, diced
- 4 beef tomatoes, toughly chopped
- 4 tbsp freshly chopped coriander
- Salt & pepper to taste

640 calories

- Place the rice in a pan of salted boiling water and cook until tender.

- Heat the oil in a frying pan and gently saute the onions & garlic for a few minutes until softened.

- Add the raisins, chicken & chopped tomatoes and continue to cook until the chicken is cooked through.

- When the chicken is cooked through add the drained rice to the pan and combine.

- Remove from the heat, stir well and serve with chopped coriander sprinkled over the top.

Feel free to toss the coriander through the dish rather than serving as a garnish if you prefer.

spinach, prawns & pinenuts

- 250g/9oz rice
- 1 tbsp olive oil
- 1 onion, chopped
- 1 tbsp freshly grated ginger
- 1 green chilli, deseeded & finely sliced
- 2 garlic cloves, crushed
- 2 tbsp lime juice
- 400g/14oz raw, peeled king prawns
- 200g/7oz spinach
- 120ml/ ½ cup chicken stock
- 3 tbsp pine nuts
- Salt & pepper to taste

405 calories

- Place the rice in a pan of salted boiling water and cook until tender.

- Heat the olive oil in a frying pan and gently saute the onions, garlic, sliced chilli & ginger for a few minutes until softened.

- Add the lime juice, prawns, spinach & stock and cook for 5-8 minutes on a high heat until the stock has reduced and the prawns are cooked through.

- Tip the drained rice into the pan along with pinenuts.

- Remove from the heat, stir well, season & serve.

If you have time, gently toast the pinenuts in a dry pan for a couple of minutes until golden brown.

thai pork kebabs & lime couscous

- 500g/1lb 2oz pork tenderloin, cubed
- 1 tbsp Thai green curry paste
- 1 tbsp coconut cream
- 1 tbsp soy sauce
- 1 lime cut into 8 wedges
- 2 onions, cut into 8 wedges each

- 370ml/1½ cups chicken stock
- 200g/7oz couscous
- 2 tbsp lime juice
- 8 kebab sticks
- Lemon wedges to serve
- Salt & pepper to taste

410 calories

- Season the pork and preheat the grill.

- Mix together the curry paste, coconut cream & soy sauce. Add the cubed pork and combine well.

- Place the pork, lime wedges and onion wedges in turn on the skewers, put under the grill and cook for 10-13 minutes or until the pork is cooked through.

- Whilst the pork is cooking, place the couscous in a pan with the hot stock and lime juice.

- Bring the pan to the boil, remove from the heat, cover and leave to stand for 3-4 minutes or until all the stock is absorbed and the couscous is tender.

- Fluff the couscous with a fork, divide onto plates and serve with the pork kebabs.

You can use any combination of vegetables you prefer with the pork to make the kebabs.

lamb kheema ghotala

- 400g/14oz lean lamb mince
- 200g/7oz rice
- 2 tbsp olive oil
- 2 onions, sliced
- 3 garlic cloves, crushed
- 2 large beef tomatoes, roughly chopped
- 2 tbsp curry powder
- 4 free range eggs
- Salt & pepper to taste

570 calories

- Place the rice in a pan of salted boiling water and cook until tender.

- Meanwhile heat the oil in a frying pan and gently saute the onions & garlic for a few minutes until softened.

- Add the tomatoes, curry powder and mince to the pan. Increase the heat and brown for 2-3 minutes.

- Reduce the heat, stir well and cook for 6-10 minutes or until the mince is cooked through.

- Whilst the rice is cooking break the eggs. Lightly beat with a fork and add to the lamb mince. Stir though to scramble for a minute or two.

- Add the drained rice and combine well. Season and serve.

For something completely different you could leave out the rice and serve this dish as a spicy Indian breakfast!

chicken & olive citrus couscous

- 500g/1lb 2oz skinless chicken breast, diced
- 1 tbsp olive oil
- 1 red pepper, deseeded & finely chopped
- 4 tbsp black pitted olives, sliced
- 2 garlic cloves, crushed
- 1 onion, sliced
- 370ml/1½ cups chicken stock
- 200g/7oz couscous
- 1 orange, juice & zest
- 1 lemon, juice & zest
- Salt & pepper to taste

495 calories

- Season the chicken.

- Gently saute the peppers, olives, garlic and onions in the olive oil for a few minutes until softened. Add the chicken to the pan and cook for 6-8 minutes or until cooked through.

- Whilst the chicken is cooking place the couscous in a saucepan with the hot stock.

- Bring the pan to the boil, remove from the heat, cover and leave to stand for 3-4 minutes or until all the stock is absorbed and the couscous is tender.

- Fluff the couscous with a fork and add to the frying pan along with the orange & lemon juice & zest.

- Toss really well and serve immediately.

Some freshly chopped mint makes a great addition to this dish.

steak & dressed greens

- 500g/1lb 2oz mini salad potatoes, quartered
- 4 sirloin steaks, each weighing 125g/4oz
- 250g/9oz spring greens

- 1 tbsp olive oil
- 1 tsp runny honey
- 1 orange, zest & juice
- Salt & pepper to taste

420 calories

- Place the potatoes and spring greens into a saucepan of salted water and cook for 6-8 minutes or until tender.

- Trim any fat off the steak, season and lightly brush with olive oil.

- Place the steak in a smoking-hot pan and cook for 1-2 minutes each side, or to your liking. When the steak is cooked, put to one side to rest for 3 minutes.

- Combine together the olive oil, honey, orange juice & zest to make a dressing.

- Drain the potatoes and greens and place in a bowl with the dressing. Season and combine well.

- Serve the steak with the dressed potatoes & greens on the side.

You could add some fresh oregano to serve with the steaks if you like.

chicken & wilted lettuce in oyster sauce

- 250g/9oz rice
- 1 tbsp olive oil
- 2 red peppers, deseeded & sliced
- 200g/7oz mushrooms, sliced

- 500g/1lb 2oz skinless chicken breasts, chopped
- 5 tbsp oyster sauce
- 2 iceberg lettuces, shredded
- Salt & pepper to taste

520 calories

- Place the rice in a pan of salted boiling water and cook until tender.

- Heat the olive oil in a frying pan or wok and gently saute the peppers and mushrooms for a few minutes until softened.

- Add the chicken and oyster sauce to the pan and fry on a high heat for 4-5 minutes or until the chicken is cooked through.

- At the end of this cooking time plunge the shredded lettuce into salted boiling water for 30 seconds.

- Add the drained rice to the pan and toss together. Season and serve immediately on top of the blanched lettuce.

Blanching the lettuce for just 30 seconds will slightly wilt the salad leaves.

sesame veggie noodles

SERVES 4

- 1 tbsp fish sauce
- 1 tbsp sesame oil
- 4 tbsp soy sauce
- 2 tbsp lime juice
- 2 tsp runny honey
- 2 tsp sesame seeds
- Salt & pepper to taste

- 2 red chillies, deseeded & finely chopped
- 4 tbsp freshly chopped coriander
- 600g/1lb 5oz straight-to-wok egg noodles

310 calories

- Mix together the fish sauce, sesame oil, soy sauce, lime juice, honey, sesame seeds & chillies to make a dressing.

- Gently warm the dressing in a saucepan and add the noodles.

- Cook for a few minutes until the noodles are piping hot.

- Divide into shallow bowls, sprinkle with chopped coriander, season & serve.

Chopped fresh basil makes a good addition to this dish too.

chicken chow mein

- 400g/14oz skinless chicken breasts
- 1 tsp Chinese 5 spice powder
- 1 tbsp olive oil
- 2 garlic cloves, crushed
- 2 carrots, cut into match sticks
- 1 onion, sliced
- 1 pointed cabbage, shredded

- 2 tbsp rice wine vinegar
- 1 tbsp fish sauce
- 3 tbsp sweet chilli sauce
- 1 tbsp soy sauce
- 250g/9oz beansprouts
- 600g/1lb 5oz straight-to-wok egg noodles
- Salt & pepper

550 calories

- Slice the chicken breast and mix with the 5 spice powder.

- Heat the olive oil in a deep sided frying pan and gently saute the garlic, carrots and onions for a few minutes until softened.

- Add the chicken and cabbage to the pan and cook for 5-7 minutes or until the chicken is cooked through.

- Mix together the rice wine vinegar, fish sauce, sweet chilli sauce and soy sauce together to make a combined sauce.

- Add the beansprouts, noodles & sauce to the pan and cook until the dish is piping hot.

- Divide into shallow bowls, season & serve.

Chopped spring onions make a perfect garnish for this dish.

pork, pineapple & peppers

- 1 tbsp olive oil
- 2 yellow peppers, deseeded & sliced
- 1 onion, sliced
- 1 red chilli, deseeded & finely chopped
- 400g/14oz pork tenderloin, diced
- 120ml/½ cup pineapple juice
- 200g/7oz pineapple chunks, drained and chopped
- 2 tbsp soy sauce
- 4 tbsp lime juice
- 600g/1lb 5oz straight-to-wok egg noodles
- 1 tbsp freshly chopped flat leaf parsley
- Salt & pepper to taste

510 calories

- Heat the olive oil in a frying pan or wok and gently saute the peppers, onions and chopped chilli for a few minutes until softened.

- Add the pork, pineapple juice, pineapple chunks, soy sauce & lime juice and continue to stir-fry until the pork is cooked through.

- Add the noodles to the pan and cook until piping hot.

- Divide into shallow bowls, sprinkle with chopped parsley & serve.

Prawns are a good alternative to pork in this recipe.

hoisin & cashew chicken stir-fry

SERVES 4

- 250g/9oz rice
- 400g/14oz skinless chicken breast
- 1 tsp runny honey
- 1 tbsp olive oil
- 1 onion, chopped
- 2 red peppers, deseeded & sliced
- 200g/7oz mangetout, trimmed
- 100g/3½oz baby sweetcorn, chopped
- 1 pak choi, shredded
- 125g/4oz cashew nuts, halved
- 2 tbsp soy sauce
- 1 tsp cornflour
- 2 tbsp hoisin sauce
- Salt & pepper to taste

620 calories

- Place the rice in a pan of salted boiling water and cook until tender.

- Cube the chicken and mix with the honey.

- Heat the olive oil in a frying pan or wok and gently saute the chopped onions, peppers, mangetout & sweetcorn for a few minutes until softened.

- Add the chicken, pak choi & nuts to the pan and cook for 4-5 minutes or until the chicken is cooked through.

- Mix together the soy sauce, cornflour and hoisin sauce to make a smooth paste (add a little water if needed). Add to the pan, turn up the heat and cook until the dish is piping hot and the chicken is cooked through..

- Add the drained rice to the pan. Combine well, season and serve immediately.

Feel free to substitute other vegetables in place of mangetout and baby corn.

chicken & noodle broth

- 200g/7oz peas
- 2 garlic cloves, crushed
- 1lt/4 cups chicken stock
- 1 tbsp freshly grated ginger
- 4 tbsp soy sauce
- 150g/5oz spinach, chopped
- 2 tbsp coconut cream

- 600g/1lb 5oz straight-to-wok egg noodles
- 400g/14oz cooked chicken breast, shredded
- 1 bunch spring onions, chopped
- Salt & pepper to taste

540 calories

- Place all the ingredients, except the chicken, coconut cream and spring onions, in a sauce pan.

- Gently cook for a 5-7 minutes. Add the shredded chicken and coconut cream, combine well and keep on the heat until the chicken is piping hot.

- Divide into four bowls and serve with the chopped spring onions sprinkled over the top.

Using cooked chicken means you can shred the meat finely before adding to the pan, which benefits the texture of the broth.

balsamic steak & rice stir-fry

- 250g/9oz rice
- 1 tbsp olive oil
- 1 red pepper, deseeded & finely sliced
- 1 onion, sliced
- 200g/7oz asparagus tips
- 200g/7oz baby sweetcorn, sliced lengthways
- 2 garlic cloves, crushed
- 2 carrots, cut into fine matchsticks
- 500g/1lb 2oz sirloin steak, thinly sliced
- 1 tbsp soy sauce
- 2 tsp runny honey
- 3 tbsp balsamic vinegar
- Salt & pepper to taste

575 calories

● Place the rice in a pan of salted boiling water and cook until tender.

● Heat the oil in a frying pan or wok and gently saute the red peppers, onions, garlic cloves, asparagus tips, baby corn and carrots for a few minutes until softened.

● Add the steak, soy sauce, honey and balsamic vinegar and cook on a high heat for 1-2 minutes.

● Add the drained rice to the pan and combine well. Season and serve.

Trim the steak of any visible fat before slicing.

lemongrass chicken thai curry

- 400g/14oz skinless, chicken breast
- 1 tbsp olive oil
- 1 onion, sliced
- 1 stalk lemongrass, finely chopped
- 1 tsp brown sugar
- 1 tbsp Thai green curry paste
- 2 tbsp lime juice
- 1 tbsp soy sauce
- 250ml/1 cup chicken stock
- 250ml/1 cup low fat coconut milk
- 600g/1lb 5oz straight-to-wok egg noodles
- 75g/3oz watercress
- Salt & pepper to taste

505 calories

- Dice & season the chicken.

- Heat the olive oil in a frying pan and gently saute the onions & lemongrass for a few minutes until softened.

- Add the chicken and cook for 4 minutes.

- Add the sugar, curry paste, lime juice, soy sauce & stock and cook for a further 2-4 minutes or until the chicken is cooked through.

- Add the noodles & coconut milk and continue to cook until the dish is piping hot.

- Divide into bowls and pile the watercress in a mound on top of each bowl.

Red Thai curry paste works just as well in this dish.

egg molee

- 250g/9oz rice
- 2 garlic cloves, crushed
- 2 onions, chopped
- 250g/9oz peas
- 1 tbsp olive oil
- 1 tsp each turmeric, garam masala & ground ginger

- 2 tbsp tomato puree
- 250ml/1 cup low fat coconut milk
- 8 large free-range hard boiled eggs
- Salt & pepper to taste

460 calories

- Place the rice in a pan of salted boiling water and cook until tender.

- Gently saute the garlic, onions & peas in the olive oil for a few minutes until softened.

- Stir through the tomato puree, dried spices & coconut milk until combined.

- Cut the eggs in half and place yolk side up, in the coconut milk. Gently cook until warmed through.

- When everything is piping hot, drain the rice and spoon the curry on top.

- Season and serve.

To hardboil the eggs; place in cold water, bring to the boil and cook for 4 mins. Remove from the heat, cool & peel.

spicy lamb & carrot burger

- 500g/1lb 2oz lean lamb mince
- 2 carrots, peeled & grated
- 2 tbsp fresh breadcrumbs
- 2 large free-range eggs
- 2 garlic cloves, crushed
- 1 tsp English mustard
- 1 tsp cumin
- 2 large plum tomatoes, sliced
- 75g/3oz watercress
- 4 wholemeal bread rolls
- Low cal cooking oil spray
- Salt & pepper to taste

580 calories

- Preheat the grill.

- Put the lamb mince, carrots, breadcrumbs, eggs, garlic, mustard & cumin in a food processor and pulse for a few seconds to combine.

- Season well and shape into four burger patties.

- Spray with a little low cal oil and place under the grill to cook for 5-6 minutes each side or until cooked through.

- Split open the rolls and when the burgers are cooked through place inside each roll.

- Lay the sliced tomatoes on top of the burger along with the watercress.

- Season and serve.

This is great served with ketchup and/or a dollop of fat free Greek yogurt.

lemon & olive penne

- 300g/11oz dried penne
- 1 tbsp olive oil
- 1 onion, sliced
- 2 garlic cloves, crushed
- 4 tbsp pitted black olives, sliced
- 1 tbsp balsamic vinegar
- 6 tbsp lemon juice
- 4 tbsp freshly chopped basil
- 200g/7oz low fat mozzarella cheese, cubed
- Salt & pepper to taste

- Cook the penne in a pan of salted boiling water until tender.

- Meanwhile heat the olive oil in a high-sided frying pan and gently saute the onions & garlic for 3-4 minutes.

- Add the olives, balsamic vinegar & lemon juice and cook until everything is tender and piping hot.

- Drain the cooked penne and add to the frying pan along with the cubed mozzarella cheese. Stir through until the cheese melts.

- Season and serve.

Make sure you serve this dish when it is still nice and hot so that the mozzarella cheese remains softly melted.

creamy parma pasta

- 1 tbsp olive oil
- 1 onion, sliced
- 200g/7oz peas
- 6 slices Parma ham, chopped
- 120ml/½ cup low fat crème fraiche
- 300g/11oz dried fusilli
- 4 tbsp freshly chopped flat leaf parsley
- 1 tbsp grated Parmesan cheese
- Salt & pepper to taste

440 calories

- Cook the fusilli and peas in a pan of salted boiling water until tender.

- Meanwhile heat the olive oil in a high-sided frying pan and gently saute the onions for a few minutes.

- When the onions are softened remove from the pan, increase the heat and add the chopped Parma ham. Cook until crispy, reduce the heat and return the onions to the pan along with the creme fraiche.

- Drain the cooked pasta and add to the frying pan along with the Parmesan cheese.

- Toss well and serve with the chopped parsley on top.

You could stir the parsley though the sauce rather than using as a garnish if you prefer.

asian chicken salad

- 1 tbsp each runny honey, soy sauce,
- olive oil & freshly grated ginger
- 2 tbsp rice wine vinegar
- 2 garlic cloves, crushed
- 500g/1lb 2oz cooked chicken breast
- ½ red chilli, deseeded & finely chopped

- 1 cucumber, sliced into batons
- 2 carrots, thinly sliced into ribbons
- 1 bunch spring onions, thinly sliced lengthways
- 1 large romaine lettuces shredded
- 4 tbsp freshly chopped coriander
- Salt & pepper to taste

280 calories

- Mix together the honey, soy sauce, olive oil, rice wine vinegar, garlic and ginger to make a dressing.

- Shred the cooked chicken. Place in a large bowl with the chilli, cucumber, carrots, spring onions and dressing. Combine well.

- Arrange the shredded lettuce on four plates and pile the dressed chicken and vegetables on top.

- Sprinkle with chopped coriander & serve.

Use a vegetable peeler to cut the carrots into very thin ribbons.

chicken & broccoli linguine

- 1 tbsp olive oil
- 2 garlic cloves, crushed
- 200g/7oz purple sprouting broccoli, roughly chopped
- 1 onion, sliced
- 300g/11oz linguine

- 400g/14oz skinless chicken breast, diced
- 1 tbsp tomato puree
- 250ml/1 cup tomato passata
- 100g/7oz rocket
- Salt & pepper to taste

520 calories

● Gently saute the garlic, broccoli, onions and chicken together in the olive oil for a few minutes in a high sided frying pan.

● Meanwhile cook the linguine in a pan of salted boiling water until tender.

● While the pasta is cooking add the tomato puree & passata to the frying pan and continue to cook until the chicken is cooked through and the broccoli is tender.

● Drain the cooked linguine and add to the pan. Stir well and, when everything is combined, quickly toss through the rocket.

● Balance the seasoning and serve immediately.

Purple sprouting broccoli is a lovely seasonal vegetable, any young tenderstem broccoli will work just as well for this recipe.

scallop sauce spaghetti

- 1 tbsp olive oil
- 1 onion, sliced
- 300g/11oz spaghetti
- 300g/11oz fresh, prepared scallops
- 60ml/¼ cup chicken stock
- 1 tbsp tomato puree
- 120ml/½ cup low fat crème fraiche
- 4 tbsp freshly chopped basil
- Salt & pepper to taste

410 calories

- Cook the spaghetti in a pan of salted boiling water until tender.

- Meanwhile gently heat the olive oil in a high-sided frying pan and saute the onion for 3-4 minutes whilst the pasta cooks. When the onions are softened add the scallops, chicken stock, tomato puree, creme fraiche & basil.

- Cook for 5 minutes or until everything is cooked through.

- Place the contents of the pan in a blender to make a smooth sauce (add a little boiling water to loosen the sauce if needed).

- Drain the pasta and toss well with the smooth scallop sauce.

- Season and serve.

Reserve a little of the basil to use as a garnish if you wish.

salmon & spanish rice

- 250g/9oz rice
- 400g/14oz skinless salmon fillets
- 2 tbsp lemon juice
- 1 tbsp olive oil
- 1 onion, sliced
- 2 garlic cloves, crushed
- 150g/5oz spinach

- 2 large beef tomatoes, roughly chopped
- 100g/3½oz chorizo, finely chopped
- 1 tsp paprika
- Salt & pepper to taste

600
calories

- Preheat the grill.

- Place the rice in a pan of salted boiling water and cook until tender.

- Brush the salmon fillets with lemon juice & a little olive oil and place under the grill. Cook for 9-12 minutes (or longer if needed) until the salmon is cooked through and flakes easily.

- Meanwhile gently saute the onions, garlic, chopped tomatoes, chorizo & paprika in a large high sided frying pan until everything softens and combines.

- Flake the cooked salmon and tip it into the saute pan along with the drained rice and spinach. Stir well until the spinach wilts.

- Season and serve.

You could pan fry the salmon if you prefer by slicing into strips and adding to the sauté pan along with the chorizo.

nepali tuna supper

- 250g/9oz rice
- 1 tbsp olive oil
- 2 onions, sliced
- 2 garlic cloves, crushed
- 1 tbsp freshly grated ginger
- 1 tbsp curry powder
- 1 tsp ground coriander
- 1 red chilli, deseeded & finely sliced
- 500g/1lb 2oz tinned tuna steak, drained
- Salt & pepper to taste

420 calories

- Place the rice in a pan of salted boiling water and cook until tender.

- Gently saute the onions and garlic in the olive oil for a 6-8 minutes until softened.

- Add the ginger, curry powder, coriander, chilli and tuna steak and cook until piping hot (add a splash of water to the pan if needed)

- When everything is piping hot tip the drained rice into the pan and combine well with the tuna and onions.

You could use fresh coriander rather than ground coriander if you have some to hand.

venison kebabs & yoghurt

- 250g/9oz rice
- 6 venison sausages
- 1 tsp each ground cumin & turmeric
- 200g/7oz ripe cherry tomatoes
- Low cal cooking oil spray

- 6 tbsp fat free Greek yoghurt
- ½ cucumber, finely chopped
- 2 tsp mint sauce
- 8 kebab skewers
- Salt & pepper to taste

440 calories

- Preheat the grill.

- Place the rice in a pan of salted boiling water and cook until tender.

- Skin the sausages and put in a food processor with the cumin and turmeric. Whizz for a few seconds to combine. Remove from the food processor and use your hands to shape into small kebab balls.

- Place the venison balls and tomatoes in turn on the skewers and spray with a little oil. Place the skewers under the grill and cook for 7-10 minutes or until cooked through.

- Mix together the yoghurt, cucumber & mint to make a raita.

- Divide the drained rice into bowls and serve with the cooked skewers on top and the minted raita on the side.

If you use wooden skewers you will need to pre-soak them in water so that they don't burn.

lime & thyme squid noodles

- 500g/1lb 2oz fresh thin squid rings
- 3 tbsp olive oil
- 2 garlic cloves, crushed
- 2 tbsp freshly chopped thyme
- 120ml/½ cup chicken stock

- 500g/1lb 2oz straight-to-wok medium noodles
- 200g/7oz peas
- 6 tbsp lime juice
- Lime wedges to serve
- Salt & pepper to taste

495 calories

- Season the squid well.

- Mix together one tablespoon of olive oil, the garlic cloves & fresh thyme to make a dressing. Combine this with the squid rings and put to one side.

- Cook the noodles and peas in the chicken stock in a saucepan until the stock reduces.

- Mix together the lime juice and the remaining two tablespoons of olive oil.

- Place the squid rings in a hot frying pan and cook for approximately 30 seconds each side, or until cooked through. Combine the fried squid, noodles & peas together along with the lime juice & olive oil.

- Toss well, season and serve.

Don't overcook the squid. 1-2 minutes of cooking should be plenty!

mustard haddock chowder

- 150g/5oz rice
- 1 tbsp olive oil
- 2 garlic cloves, crushed
- 1 onion, sliced
- 2 carrots, diced
- 150g/5oz potatoes, diced
- 1 tsp turmeric
- 1 tsp English mustard

- 500ml/2 cups semi skimmed milk
- 400g/14oz boneless, skinless smoked haddock fillets, cubed
- 4 tbsp freshly chopped flat leaf parsley
- Salt & pepper to taste

370 calories

- Place the rice in a pan of salted boiling water and cook until tender.

- Gently saute the garlic, onions, carrots & potatoes for a few minutes until softened.

- Add the turmeric, mustard, milk & haddock. Cover and leave to gently poach for 8-10 minutes or until the fish is cooked through and the vegetables are tender.

- Add the drained rice to the milk pan.

- Combine well, season and serve with parsley sprinkled over the top.

This is a really hearty chowder. You can make it go a little further by adding additional milk.

watercress gnocchi

SERVES 4

- 1 tbsp olive oil
- 1 tsp crushed garlic
- 1 onion, sliced

- 700g/1lb 9oz gnocchi
- 400g/14oz watercress
- 2 tbsp truffle oil
- Salt & pepper to taste

350 calories

- Gently saute the garlic and onions in the olive oil for a few minutes

- Whilst the onions are softening place the gnocchi in a pan of salted boiling water. Cook for 2-3 minutes or until the gnocchi begins to float to the top.

- Meanwhile plunge the watercress into a fresh pan of boiling water and blanch for one minute. Drain and refresh immediately with cold water.

- As soon as the gnocchi is cooked, drain and place in the frying pan with everything else.

- Turn the heat up and move the gnocchi around for a few minutes to coat each dumpling in the truffle oil and garlic and combine with the wilted watercress.

- Check the seasoning and serve.

Serve with some grated Parmesan or Pecorino cheese if you like.

jamaican chicken salad

300 calories

SERVES 4

- 500g/1lb 2oz skinless chicken breast
- 2 tsp crushed chilli flakes,
- 4 tbsp lime juice
- 1 tsp mixed spice
- 1 tbsp olive oil
- 1 onion, sliced

- 6 large plum tomatoes, roughly chopped
- 1 red pepper, deseeded & sliced
- 300g/11oz mixed salad leaves
- Salt & pepper to taste

- Season the chicken and slice into thin strips.

- Mix together the chilli flakes, lime juice, mixed spice and olive oil in a bowl to make a dressing.

- Add the chicken slices to the bowl and combine well.

- Gently saute the dressed chicken, onions, tomatoes and peppers in the pan (add a little more oil if needed).

- When the chicken is cooked through arrange on a bed of mixed salad leaves to serve.

This dish is good served with some fat free natural yoghurt to balance the heat of chilli.

sweet & spicy steak salad

350 calories

- 500g/1lb 2oz sirloin steak
- 2 tbsp olive oil
- 2 tsp runny honey
- 1 tbsp ketchup
- 1 tbsp soy sauce
- 3 tbsp lime juice
- ½ tsp crushed chilli flakes
- 4 large plum tomatoes, chopped
- 300g/11oz mixed spinach and rocket leaves
- 1 red onion, finely sliced
- Salt & pepper to taste

- Trim any fat off the steak and lightly brush with a little of the olive oil. Season and slice into strips before putting a frying pan on a high heat.

- Place the steak strips in the smoking-hot pan and cook for 1-2 minutes .

- Reduce the heat and add the rest of the olive oil, honey, ketchup, soy sauce, lime juice and chilli flakes.

- Combine really well and cook for a minute or two longer.

- Arrange the chopped tomatoes, salad leaves and red onion onto plates and place the sliced steak strips on top.

- Season and serve.

Adjust the cooking time depending on how you wish your steak to be cooked.

lemon & oregano tuna steaks

SERVES 4

- 1 garlic clove, crushed
- 4 tbsp olive oil
- 2 tbsp lemon juice
- 4 tbsp freshly chopped oregano
- 4 fresh tuna steaks, each weighing 150g/5oz

- 200g/7oz cherry tomatoes, halved
- 1 red onion, sliced
- 150g/5oz watercress
- Salt & pepper to taste

305 calories

- Mix together the garlic, olive oil, lemon juice & oregano in a bowl to make a dressing. Use a little of the dressing to brush on either side of the tuna steak. Place the halved tomatoes and sliced onions in the bowl with the rest of the dressing and coat well.

- Put the tomatoes and red onions in a pan and saute for 2-4 minutes. Mix together the garlic, olive oil, lemon juice & oregano in a bowl to make a dressing. Use a little of the dressing to brush on either side of the tuna steak. Place the halved tomatoes and sliced onions in the bowl with the rest of the dressing and coat well.

- Put the tomatoes and red onions in a pan and saute for 2-4 minutes. Whilst the tomatoes are cooking, place the tuna steak under a preheated medium grill and cook for 2-3 minutes each side or until the tuna is cooked to your liking.

- Remove the tuna from the grill and serve with the onions and tomatoes piled on top and the watercress on the side.

The tomatoes and onions should be warmed through but still have a little crunch to them.

pea & parmesan risotto

- 2 tbsp olive oil
- 1 garlic clove, crushed
- 1 onion, sliced
- 1 celery stalk, finely chopped
- 300g/11oz Arborio risotto
- 400g/7oz peas

- 1lt/4 cups vegetable stock/ broth
- 1 tbsp fresh grated Parmesan cheese
- Salt & pepper to taste

420 calories

- Heat the olive oil and gently saute the garlic, onion & celery for a few minutes until softened.

- Add the risotto rice to the pan and stir well to coat each grain in olive oil. Add a ladle of stock and simmer until the stock is absorbed. Continue cooking the risotto adding a ladle of stock each time and allowing the rice to absorb the stock until adding the next ladle.

- Continue cooking for about 15 minutes or until the rice is tender. Add more stock if needed and continue the process until tender.

- Meanwhile add the peas to boiling water and cook for 4-5 minutes or until tender. Add the drained peas to the pan and stir through the grated Parmesan cheese.

- Season & serve.

Risotto is traditionally made using white wine. Try substituting ¼ of the stock with wine if you like!

greek chicken kebabs

- 2 garlic cloves, crushed
- 1lt/4 cups chicken stock
- 1 tbsp olive oil
- 2 tsp dried oregano
- 3 tbsp lemon juice

- 500g/1lb 2oz skinless chicken breasts, cubed
- 200g/7oz rice
- Salt & pepper to taste
- Metal skewers

420 calories

- Preheat the grill to a medium/high heat.

- Mix together the garlic, olive oil, oregano & lemon juice in a bowl.

- Season the chicken and add to the bowl. Combine well and skewer each piece to make four large chicken kebabs.

- Place under the grill and cook for 6-8 minutes each side or until the chicken is cooked through and piping hot.

- Meanwhile cook the rice in the chicken stock until tender.

- Remove the kebabs from the grill, season and serve with the drained rice.

You could add some chopped vegetables to the rice and serve with a little fat free Greek yoghurt on the side if you wish.

94

cavalfiori risotto

- 1 large cauliflower head
- 2 tbsp olive oil
- 2 garlic cloves, crushed
- 1 onion, sliced
- 1 celery stalk, finely chopped
- 300g/11oz Arborio risotto

- 1lt/4 cups vegetable stock/ broth
- 4 tbsp freshly chopped flat leaf parsley
- Salt & pepper to taste

370 calories

- Break up the cauliflower head into florets and place in a food processor. Pulse until the cauliflower turns into rice sized grains.

- Heat the olive oil and gently saute the onion, celery and garlic for a few minutes until softened.

- Add the risotto rice to the pan and stir well to coat each grain in olive oil. Add a ladle of stock and simmer until the stock is absorbed. Add the cauliflower to the pan.

- Continue cooking the risotto adding a ladle of stock each time and allowing the rice to absorb the stock until adding the next ladle. This should take about 15-20 minutes. Add more stock if needed and continue to cook until tender.

- Season and serve with chopped parsley.

'Cavalfioro' or 'cauliflower' risotto is a popular creamy risotto dish in Italy.

fennel & chickpea chicken

- 1 tbsp olive oil
- 1 onion, sliced
- 1 celery stalk, finely chopped
- 2 carrots, diced
- 1 fennel bulb, finely sliced
- 1 tsp fennel seeds, crushed
- 3 garlic cloves, crushed
- 300g/11oz tinned chickpeas, drained
- 500g/1lb 2oz skinless chicken breasts, thickly sliced
- 120ml/½ cup chicken stock
- Salt & pepper to taste

380 calories

- Gently saute the onion, celery, carrots, fennel, fennel seeds & garlic in the olive oil for a few minutes until softened.

- Add the chickpeas, chicken & stock and leave to gently simmer for 10-15 minutes or until the chicken is cooked through, the stock has reduced and the carrots are tender.

- Season and serve.

You could serve this as a thick broth: add more stock and pulse for a few seconds in a blender or food processor.